# Living With Lung and Colon Endometriosis

# Catamenial Pneumothorax

By

Glynis D. Wallace D.M.D.

authorHOUSE™

1663 Liberty Drive, Suite 200
Bloomington, Indiana 47403
(800) 839-8640
www.AuthorHouse.com

*First published by AuthorHouse 09/20/05*

*ISBN: 1-4208-8328-3 (e)*
*ISBN: 1-4208-8331-3 (sc)*

*Library of Congress Control Number: 2005908052*

*Printed in the United States of America*
*Bloomington, Indiana*

*This book is printed on acid-free paper.*

## Dedication

I dedicate this book in memory of my wonderful mother Martha N. Robinson, who was by my side through every surgery praying for me.

## Acknowledgements

I would like to thank the United States Air force (Wilford Hall Medical Center), Army (Tripler Army Hospital), and Navy (Balboa Navy Medical Center). I am profoundly grateful for the wonderful medical care rendered and sparing no expense to diagnose and treat my Catamenial Pneumothoracies.

# Contents

# Introduction

I wrote this book to share information and enlighten the nation about pulmonary endometriosis. Pulmonary refers to the lung. Endometriosis refers to tissue from the mucous membrane of the uterus where females carry their babies. Endometrial implants appear on the lung like chocolate cysts and release blood between the lung and its lining, which is known as the pleura. Menstruation, monthly flow of blood, occurring on the lung every month is a strange reality and difficult concept to fathom. This phenomenon, known as catamenial hemopneumothorax, is when endometriosis attaches to the lung, releases fluid, and allows air to move in by an unknown mechanism—all of which causes the lung to collapse. For several years, denial was my coping mechanism, but after three major surgeries to remove endometriosis, seven chest tube operations to inflate and remove fluid from my lung, and extensive research, I conceded to the humbling reality. Many medical professionals do not know about this syndrome and most standard textbooks do not mention it. The literature states that 100 people in the U.S. have this rare gynecological disease, but the truth is only 100 appear in the literature. I am convinced, along with my pulmonologist and gynecologist, that many women go undiagnosed due to lack of knowledge in the medical world. I hope my story helps others suffering with this strange yet maybe not so rare disease. Although the U.S. has only 100 recorded cases, there are millions of women all over the world who suffer from the pain and infertility caused by endometriosis.

This book outlines my 13-year experience with pulmonary endometriosis through narrative summaries from the physicians who attempted to control this disease. As an active duty military officer, I underwent extensive and extremely thorough diagnostic tests to determine fitness for duty. This led to excellent medical treatment, which allowed me to continue serving on active duty. . I would like to thank the military, Air Force,

Army, and Navy—all of whom I owe my life for sparing no expense to treat the disease and keep me alive over the years.

# Chapter 1
# Symptoms and Initial Diagnosis

I was a relatively healthy child, hospitalized once at age twelve for a bruised kidney after a bicycle accident.

After graduating from Westchester High School in 1974, I earned a Bachelor of Science degree from California State University–Long Beach and entered the medical world of cancer research, where many chemicals used for invitro studies with mice were later ruled out as a causative agent for my disease. I moved on to graduate school and earned a Doctor of Medical Dentistry degree from Tufts University School of Dental Medicine. After graduation, I worked as a dental associate before entering the United States Public Health Service (USPHS)–Federal Bureau of Prisons as a commissioned officer.

On Monday, July 29, 1991 the first symptoms occurred. I felt a mild pain on the lower right just below my rib cage near the diaphragm, and had trouble breathing when lying flat. I also experienced slight shortness of breath with exertion and coughing while running.

I lived in Big Spring, Texas, serving as an active duty Lieutenant in the USPHS detailed to the Federal Bureau of Prisons. Working in the prison had required extensive training, exercise and long hours, and I had recently returned from a self-defense course where I was taught with physical vigor. This is my first recollection of the dull pain that would resurface every month.

My mother lived in Midland, Texas, about 35 miles away. After discussing my symptoms with her, I made an appointment at a small clinic for an ultrasound to rule out a possible gall stone, which I thought was causing my lower right side pain, since the liver and gallbladder are located right under the diaphram. The ultrasound revealed that my abdomen was full of fluid, which was strange because my stomach was flat. The physician decided that an ovarian malignancy was possibly causing the fluid and notified the USPHS who immediately arranged transport to one of the best military medical centers in the world. I was not aware of his initial suspicions, but the quick move-to-action by the USPHS told me it was possibly more serious than I initially thought.

The next day, I was medvaced to Wilford Hall, United States Air Force Medical Center. Upon arrival I had a chest X-ray, which revealed 3400 cubic centimeters (cc) of fluid on my right lung. The radiology team seemed to be peeking around the corner at me, giving me cause for alarm, so to calm my nerves I began to pray. After what seemed like an eternity, I was admitted and taken to my room where my team came by for an introduction before leaving for the day. That night, one of the residents (who later became my guardian angel) removed 1650 cc of fluid from my right lung by thoracentesis—puncturing the chest wall to let liquids out of the chest cavity—making a small dent in its appearance on the postoperative X-ray. The red fluid seemed to impress him, and he informed me that the pathologist would give us results as soon as possible.

The next day, a team of colorectal surgeons who specialize in operating on the colon and rectum of the bowel came in to inform me that I possibly had lupus; however, more tests were required for a diagnosis. You will find out later how it was fate that they accepted me as a patient on their service. The ultrasound was repeated the next day and a series of pulmonary tests were initiated.

A couple of days passed and the pathologist could not make a definitive diagnosis from the fluid, so the surgical resident who previously removed 1650cc's of fluid attempted to remove the rest of it, but not without incident. I remember joking with the surgical resident in reference to what side he would be inserting the tube, right or left and making the comment that he had great hands and should have been a surgeon. He grinned and said, "touché." I would have never guessed in the next five minutes that my world would change dramatically.

My head felt like it would explode as I went into shock and actually saw the proverbial bright light up and off to the right. I remember sitting upright and feeling a strange pressure in the brain stem area and then around my heart, causing my body to go limp with perfuse perspiration. But my eyes were drawn to the light. I had heard about the light followed by a tunnel before, but was not sure I actually believed it. My family had flown in for support and my mother stood in the doorway, watching as my blood pressure and pulse began to drop and I drifted into shock. Her nursing instincts must have taken over because she ran to my bedside to help, and the last thing I remember was her voice saying, "70/40 and pulse 42." I woke up with my team standing over me, informing me I would be moved to a different floor.

Exhausted after the experience, I went back to sleep and woke to the voice of a physician asking me if I knew what had happened to me. Discussing the incident of the bright light helped as I attempted to rationalize the experience. The surgeons thought it was due to the severity of the vaso-vagal reflex, commonly known as syncope (temporary loss of consciousness due to deficiency of blood carrying oxygen to the brain). No, I knew this was different from syncope and did not except that explanation, leading me to believe I was in real trouble and it was time for prayer and faith—I was taught the bigger your problems, the bigger your prayers have to be. My family was allowed in and helped me stay strong. Somehow, the most memorable occurrence during my hospitalization was not included in my narrative summary.

There was one short statement about it in my medical record, which told me the surgeons considered it to be somewhat insignificant.

Many tests were ordered over the next several days, but I was allowed to leave the hospital after my IV was removed or heparin locked. And of course, duty hours were over, so I was able to see some of San Antonio with my family. This was good except my team had the messenger-of-misery look on their faces, which radiated an impending feeling of doom. To enhance this look, a CA 125 blood test for ovarian cancer was ordered. This test determines the level of antigen in the blood known to be a tumor marker, and it also detects some benign conditions like endometriosis in the abdomen and chest. The normal range for CA 125 is 0-35 and my test revealed a high level of 85, meaning there was a 1% chance my diagnosis was endometriosis.

The next two weeks presented a medical adventure that was both puzzling because the diagnosis had eluded my doctors and exciting because reinforcements from every specialty had been called in. None of the tests conclusively rendered a diagnosis that would allow us to start on a cure, but my spirituality kept me strong.

As a doctor who's been on the other side, I had a difficult time accepting the rude awakening of a consult, something that no longer meant a talk with the specialist, but rather a painful, invasive procedure required to collect information.

Pulmonary specialists requested tests for tuberculosis and every other type of lung disease they could think of; all came back with negative results. The Air Force spared no expense ordering ultrasounds, cat scans, upper endoscopy procedures and lower colonoscopy procedures (when the inside of the colon is examined). The colonoscopy did not yield the information needed to make a diagnosis, so the specialists did another colon test; called a contrast barium enema, and they finally saw a large mass pressing from the outside. More confirmation came from the urology department where I was sent for a cystoscopy to have the inside of my bladder examined. The test revealed a mass poking in from the back, so now I had several masses in my abdomen and a lot of fluid on my lung.

During the entire testing period, I felt fine, so I continued my tours of San Antonio. The river walk down there is beautiful and it gave me an opportunity to get away from the sadness I saw in the staff's eyes.

They didn't share all the information with me; every day I would grab my record from the nurse's station, so I could keep up and maybe stay one step ahead of them. When I read they had consulted with and were referring me to GYN Oncology, my world fell apart. With all my faith and so many people praying, how could I have cancer and how would it have moved from my abdomen to my lung with no pain and sickness? They had to be wrong, and I had to find out right away if they were.

An extremely positive resident, who had always taken the opportunity to tell me I looked too good to have cancer, informed me that the head of general surgery did not like to have active duty people lying around for a long time and that I should talk to him about doing exploratory surgery to find out what was going on. It was time for a move to action with aggressive treatment, since I believe physicians treat and God heals, treatment in some form needed to start immediately. Being assertive at that point was my best option or it could have dragged on for a while. So after a lot of tears, I got out of my bed and walked down to GYN Oncology to find the doctor my team had consulted with and asks him if he thought I had cancer, since it wasn't clearly written on my record. The gentle soul I met was a nice, caring doctor whose name eludes me now, and he told me that if I arranged the surgery for the next day, he would be in the operating room so we could find out. I guess he saw and felt my desperation. With that commitment from Gyn Oncology, I was ready to give the colorectal surgeons the information when they made their rounds. They immediately began to prepare me for the laparoscopy/laparatomy scheduled for the next day at 5:00 am. They wanted to find out what it was as much as I did.

There were many pre-surgical preparations required for what physically would change my life forever, but the most important preparations for me were mental. I wanted a son and wasn't sure if a hysterectomy would be performed, but knew it was a possibility. If they did find cancer, what would the next step be? My first thought: if it was cancer and I made it out of there, there was no way I was paying back all those student loans from dental school. Maybe I was a little confused, and it was a good thing my family was there to help me focus. We all decided it was time to get in touch with a master physician who could provide healing and health restoration. This would increase my faith and help me stay positive to enhance the possibility of an optimal outcome. I had a lot of fear and we wanted it to stand for False Evidence Appearing Real.

# Chapter 2

## First Surgery with the Air Force and Narrative Summary

I was taken to the operating room on 16 Aug 1991 at 0500 where I underwent a diagnostic laparoscopy/laparotomy, commonly known as exploratory surgery. Present in the operating room were representatives from Colorectal Surgery, General Surgery, Pulmonary Medicine and GYN Oncology. Two sections of my colon were removed with a frozen section that was sent to Pathology during the surgery, confirming endometriosis. As the saying goes, "tissue is the issue"! Pulmonary checked for endometriosis leading to my lung under the diaphragm and found nothing conclusive. GYN Oncology checked the reproductive system and found no endometriosis attached, so a hysterectomy was not performed and the opportunity to have a child was preserved.

I will never forget the specialists' expressions when they woke me up and told me they had found endometriosis attached to my colon and that nobody ever died from endometriosis. Bewilderment, shock and relief showed in their eyes. I thought I was safe, but a few days later the same pain I had on the right returned. A chest X-ray revealed the fluid on my lung had returned as well. GYN informed me I would be given a shot of an intramuscular medication called Lupron Depot (leuprolide acetate for depot suspension). Lupron Depot belongs to a class of drugs called gonadotropin-releasing hormone (GnRH) agonists. It works to manage endometriosis by lowering hormone levels and that decreases Endometrial growths and provides relief of symptoms. Lupron Depot is available as an injection and would be given once a month for 6 months to treat the fluid on my lung, and if this didn't work, I would need more surgery. I was discharged from the hospital and allowed to go home for one month.

When I returned to the hospital two months later, a chest X-ray revealed all fluid had disappeared, leading me to believe I was cured. My instructions were to complete a six-month course of Lupron Depot.

Lupron Depot (leuprolide acetate for depot suspension) decreases the body's production of specific hormones. By decreasing estrogen, it reduces the endometriotic lesions causing pain relief. Because Lupron Depot can reduce the production of both male and female hormones, it is used to treat prostate cancer in men, endometriosis and fibroids in women and precocious puberty in children. It belongs to a class of drugs called gonadotropin-releasing hormone (GnRH) agonists.

I took one 3.75 mg-shot per month for a 6-month period, causing me to have extreme hot flashes, which I controlled with soy milk. Other side effects included headaches and vaginal dryness. Bone loss can also occur during therapy with Lupron Depot, but in most cases it returns to normal after therapy stops.

## NARRATIVE SUMMARY

DATE OF ADMISSION: 30 JULY 91
DATE OF DISCHARGE: 28 AUG 91

INTRODUCTION: This is a 34-year-old black female dentist in the public health service who presents to WHMC with abdominal pain and shortness of breath times two weeks.

HISTORY OF PRESENT ILLNESS: The patient reports a two-week history of progressive shortness of breath and right upper quadrant pain, which is dull and aching in character with radiation to her right shoulder, and progressing to a very intense aching type pain in the right upper quadrant several days prior to admission. She also reported three-pillow orthopnea for the couple of weeks prior to admission as well as shortness of breath and dyspnea on exertion. The patient reports the pain initially started approximately three months prior to admission but had resolved over the ensuing period. The patient reports having had intermittent bouts of anemia for approximately two months. She denies any nausea, hematemesis, acholic stools, hematochezia, melena or history of jaundice. The patient reports a history of lactose intolerance, and occasional episodes of right-sided chest pain, which was relieved with Alka-Seltzer. She notes the pain in her upper right quadrant becomes worse with eating, approximately 30 minutes to several hours postprandially. The patient's GYN history is remarkable for episodes of menstrual pain, and she states her menses are expected to start the day after admission.

Past History: Social history: remarkable for no tobacco use, no drug abuse, and occasional social drinking of alcohol. Family history is remarkable for a history of breast cancer and uterine cancer in female members of the family. The patient's past medical history is remarkable only for a history of iron deficiency anemia for which she was treated with iron sulfate orally. Previous injuries include a kidney injury secondary to fall at age 12, without any sequelae. The patient reports no known drug allergies.

Review of Systems: Remarkable only for heavy four-day periods. 35 days in the menstrual cycle, with occasional menstrual pain without breakthrough bleeding or pain between cycles.

PHYSICAL EXAMINATION: Demonstrated a well-developed black female in no apparent distress. Vital signs were normal and her temperature was 97.8 degrees orally.

HEENT: unremarkable. Chest was symmetric and non-tender, and examination of the breast demonstrated no skin changes or dimpling with clear fluid expressible from both nipples and diffuse fibrocystic changes. Lungs demonstrated decreased breath sounds at the right base with dullness to percussion approximately half way up the right lung field, but were otherwise clear to auscultation.

Cardiac examination demonstrated regular rate and rhythm without murmurs, bruits, or JVD. Examination of the abdomen demonstrated a soft flat abdomen with normal bowel sounds throughout, non-tender, with deep 2-3 cm fullness in the right periumbilical region. The pelvic and rectal exams demonstrated normal external female genitalia without lesions or discharge and an unremarkable bimanual examination with normal rectal tone, no masses, and heme negative. Examination of the extremities demonstrated no lesions or tenderness.

LABORATORY AND X-RAY DATA: WBC 6.8, hematocrit of 36.6, platelets 351,000 PT/PTT 13/29.2. Sodium 142, potassium 4.1, chloride 106, CO2 24, BUN 8, creatinine 0.9, glucose 75, calcium 8.7, phosphorus 3.8, total bilirubin 0.6, alkaline phosphatase 64, AST 10, LDH 188, albumin 4.1. UA demonstrated 10-14 red cells, 1-4 epithelial cells, trace ketones. Chest X-ray demonstrated an obvious fluid collection in the right lung space with collapsed lobe of the lung.

HOSPITAL COURSE: The patient was admitted to the General Surgery Service for workup of a spontaneous right pleural effusion and shortness of breath with non-specific abdominal complaints. Thoracentesis of the right chest produced 1650 cc of chocolate brown thin fluid, cytology of which was remarkable only for copious red blood and benign mesothelial cells. After drainage of the right pleural effusion, the patient had relief of her symptoms for several days, however, continued to complain of diffuse abdominal discomfort. A pelvic ultrasound demonstrated no evidence of adenexal mass or cyst, with ovaries not well visualized, with a small amount of ascites. A pelvic and abdominal CT was also obtained, which demonstrated a small right pleural effusion, mild to moderate ascites, no definite ovarian mass, and a 2 cm small uterine fibroid. Subsequently, upper and lower endoscopy was attempted to rule out any GI source of pathology. Upper endoscopy demonstrated a slight amount of distal esophagitis as well as a less than 5 mm mucosal abnormality high in the fundus, benign appearing. Colonoscopy was attempted, however, due to redundant amount of sigmoid colon, a C-scope was unable to be passed. Subsequent to this, an aircontrast barium enema was obtained, with findings reported to be extrinsic compression of the cecum without other masses or lesions. At the same time, an anergy panel had been placed without reaction to inciting controlled test. By this time, Pulmonary Medicine,

Internal Medicine, and GYN Service had been consulted. Given the patient's employment in the Texas State Prison System and the incidence of TB in the working environment, the possibility of a mycobacterial infection could not be excluded from the diagnosis and hence the patient was sent for induced sputum samples times three days, the results of which primarily demonstrated no AFB in the sputum samples. In addition, the patient also reported a history several months prior to admission of performing tae kwon do, with subsequent chest trauma from the exercise, and so Medicine recommended obtaining a routine ventilation profusion scan to rule out any pulmonary vascular insults. This procedure was reported as low probability for pulmonary embolus. Repeat UA from the initial admission UA was remarkable for 1-4 RBCs per high power field and subsequently Urology was consulted as well to workup the possibility of UT involvement. Subsequently, a cystoscopy demonstrated normal bladder mucosa and normal ureteral orifices bilaterally with an extrinsic mass posteriorly in the midline, which did not move with cervical motion. Bilateral retrogrades demonstrated no obvious lesions, and a cyctogram was unremarkable. Also obtained as part of the laboratory workup was a CEA, which was 2.8

(normal) and a CA125 which was elevated at 85. Quantitative HCG was negative, HIV was negative, and ANA was negative at less than 1:180. TFT's were remarkable for a T4 of 9.3, T3RU 28, all within normal limits. Rheumatoid factor was noted to be equivocally positive. Amylase was normal at 110. Given the patient's persistence of symptoms with slow recurrence of the right pleural effusion (although this time without symptoms), and a consultation with the Pulmonary and GYN Oncology Services, the patient was taken to the OR on 16 Aug 91 where she underwent a diagnostic laparoscopy/laparotomy/segmental resection of transverse colon with sewn anastomosis/ illocecal resection with end to side anastomosis. Findings intraoperatively on frozen section demonstrated endometriosis, with dark pelvic fluid consistent with old blood (approximately 150 cc) noted deep in the pelvis, a subserosal 1.5 cm mass at the cecum with endometrial implants, and subserosal mass at the distal transverse colon. The patient tolerated the procedure well, and her postoperative course was only remarkable for a slow recovery of bowel function. On postoperative day #8, the patient was tolerating sips of clear liquids and by postoperative day #10, she was tolerating a regular diet. Postoperatively, a chest x-ray as well as decubitus films were obtained, which showed recurrence of the fluid collection with minimal symptoms at that time. Of note, the patient was due to begin her next menstrual cycle, and noted the onset of right sided chest discomfort and right chest discomfort similar to her symptoms prior to presentation, consistent with the progressive right pleural effusion. Given the diagnosis of endometriosis, the patient was placed on intramuscular Lupron Depot Q. month and is to be followed by GYN Service over the next several months to monitor response.

CONSULTATIONS:

1. GYN Oncology
2. Pulmonary Medicine
3. Internal Medicine
4. Urology

OPERATIONS AND PROCEDURES: See hospital course

FINAL DIAGNOSIS:
1. Extrapelvic endometriosis

LINE OF DUTY: Yes

DISPOSITION AND/OR RECOMMENDATION: The patient is discharged to home with con leave and profile. Medications on discharge include: Percocet (#20/Tylenol ES), MOM/ Metamucil. The patient is to follow-up with the GYN Service as directed and the Pulmonary Service as well approximately three weeks after discharge, and she is to follow-up with the General Surgery Service as needed for abdominal complaints of signs or symptoms of infection in the wound.

APPROVED:

# Chapter 3

## Seven Years Symptom Free

Having no pain and no symptoms, in my mind, was a real miracle and just one of many to appear over the next few years of coping with this disease. After a few weeks of rest and recuperation, I had a favorable follow-up visit because the fluid on my lung had resolved and I was released. You see, at this point in my life I did not know there was no cure for endometriosis. Continuing the expensive medication ($500 dollars a shot) for six months made me feel great health wise. I wasn't aware that Lupron Depot does not destroy the endometriol cells, but only suppresses and inhibits their secretion or bleeding.

My faith restored, I went back to Midland. The next week, my grandmother, one of my main prayer warriors, had a cerebral stroke after telling me she had asked God to take her if he needed someone and to allow me to stay here and be "a help to the nation." This expression has become a theme for me in my family. As an infant, a minister had prayed that I would some day be a help to the nation. Writing this book to deliver information about pulmonary endometriosis should satisfy that.

After my grandmother's funeral, the USPHS transferred me to California and I continued care with the GYN department at March Air Force Base in Moreno Valley, CA. Finishing the six months of Lupron Depot, I transitioned onto birth control pills—ortho novum 1/35—to keep the endometriosis from coming back.

My position in California was with the Federal Bureau of Prisons on Terminal Island. Different from the smaller prison in Big Spring, Texas, this one had towers manned by correctional officers with guns; there were many high-profile federal inmates here. My commander was very nice and extremely happy I had joined him to offer dental treatment to inmates. We were the only two dentists, with one civilian assistant and two inmate dental-assistant trainees.

The transition was fairly smooth since I was allowed to live at the Long Beach Naval Station for two months. My goal was to recover quickly and put the sickness behind me as soon as possible. I was in great shape and received an award for outstanding performance in self-defense in 1992. This is also where I met the love of my life. A kind, understanding physician serving in the USPHS, he briefly assumed temporary duty at the prison. He wanted children, and I was happier than ever a hysterectomy had not been performed.

That year, I also left the USPHS to pursue a private-practice opportunity, which is every dentist's dream. Although I enjoyed the experience, my student loans were overwhelming. I kept in touch with friends in the USPHS and found an offer I couldn't refuse: loan repayment if I went to work on an isolated Indian reservation with the Navajos in Arizona. Dental school was extremely expensive, so this seemed to be an attractive way to pay off student loans and have a great adventure. There had been no problems with my health, and the vigorous physical I underwent to go back on active duty confirmed my miraculous cure. My lungs were clear of abnormalities.

In November 1993 I arrived in Tsaile Arizona on the Navajo nation, 85 miles one way from the closest McDonald's and Wal-Mart, located in Gallup, New Mexico. There was a clinic, 20 government houses and a trading post, and the land and countryside was beautiful. The Navajos were the nicest, most easygoing and appreciative patients I will have ever treated. My only illness during this isolated, one-year hardship tour on the reservation was a bile blockage, which was resolved without hospitalization. It was probably due to adhesions in the GI tract from the previous colon surgery. I hiked through Canyon de Shey, played snow volleyball, and worked very hard as Chief Dental Officer of the Tsaile Clinic. I was intrigued with the spirituality surrounding the medicine man and how much influence he had on the Navajo nation. It was truly a unique experience.

After the year ended, I was detailed back to the Federal Bureau of Prisons in Greenville, Illinois. For the first two weeks, I lived at Scott Air Force Base where I met several members of the Air Force medical and dental staff. Although I remained in good health and without limitations or symptoms, I would now receive medical care from these professionals. I settled into my new position and participated in annual training, which consisted of self-defense, riot control and other law enforcement activities. It paid off when a prison riot occurred and ten hostages were taken. This real-world situation gave me the opportunity to use the security knowledge I had obtained and to increase my suturing skills while providing care for the wounded.

A decision to leave the USPHS after the riot led me to pursue a career in the United States Air Force (USAF). The people I met at Scott AFB told me about the wonderful experiences and travel opportunities available. I had never been out of the U.S., so this was my opportunity, not to mention the safest and least expensive method to see the world. The Air Force accepted me right away, and on April 22, 1997, I was on my way to Commissioned Officer Training in Montgomery, Alabama at Gunter Air Force Base (AFB) to become an officer in the USAF. After settling in, I was informed that due to my prior experience in the USPHS, which they were impressed with, I had been selected as Student Operations Group Commander for the other 120 Commissioned Officer Training attendees. I would help orchestrate the groups move from place to place. It was exciting and different from anything I had ever experienced—I was in the real military now. United States Public Health Service is one of the seven uniformed services, with 4800 officers (Medical and Dental).

In Commissioned Officer Training, we were taught how to march, salute, wear uniforms correctly, use military courtesy and everything else that would make us effective, efficient officers. We ran a mile a day and I had no signs or symptoms of any pulmonary distress.

Life was good and I had found my place. I climbed over walls using ropes and it was fun and exciting. The training ended, and I became a full-pledged military officer. After graduation, I would leave to fulfill my duties in Osan, South Korea.

This would be my first time out of the United States. It was an incredible new adventure that allowed me to travel in a foreign country and be introduced to new foods and a new culture. The military aspect was not bad either, except for the exercises with a flap jacket, kevlar helmet, chemical gear (which weighed fifty pounds), and of course the dreaded gas mask. The camaraderie was outstanding and I developed great friendships I will cherish for a lifetime.

# Chapter 4
# Collapsed Lung

After the third exercise, I found out that my lung condition did not agree with wearing the gas mask and the breathing resistance had taken its toll. In January 1998 it began to feel cold in my chest while inhaling. I had never had pneumonia, but I thought it was a possibility since it was twenty degrees outside and covered with snow and ice. One of the physician's assistants working in the primary care clinic listened to my lungs and didn't hear any sounds on the lower right. He ordered a chest X-ray, which revealed a pneumothorax at the apex of the right lung. I couldn't believe it, and since I was not in any real distress except for the cold feeling I had in my chest, I decided not to allow a chest tube to be placed. It was about 11:00 am in the morning when I went home and ate lunch, then came back and all hell broke loose.

The general surgeon chased me around, attempting to explain the importance of putting in a chest tube immediately. One of the internal medicine docs, a close friend, joined forces with the surgeons, and after several hours of resisting I was admitted to the Osan hospital, where I worked, and my first chest tube was placed. I phoned my mother in Midland, Texas just before I was taken to the operating room to let her know what was happening. The anesthesia kept me groggy for several hours, while my mother called the Red Cross, who came through for her after she had found the original second half of my social security card in her bible, enabling her to give them the number so they could track me through the military locator. This was a spiritual sign that I would be all right.

I woke up with a chest tube protruding from my side and hooked up to wall suction, accompanied by a lot of pain. After a few days, it was evident a resolution of the pneumothorax had not occurred and an additional chest tube would be required. I was asked if I would allow other doctors to observe the placement of the second chest tube so they would be proficient in wartime. As a member of the hospital staff, I had considered it my opportunity to offer more service to my colleagues and the military, so I agreed. At that time, I would have never guessed how many more opportunities I would have in the next few years to participate in chest tube-placement demonstration. It was back to the operating room, where an additional chest tube was placed in a strategic spot right at the apex of my lung. Unfortunately, the second chest tube did not resolve the problem either.

My military family was there to keep me strong and positive. We had parties in my hospital room and there was always someone dropping by just to keep me company. It was great and I really appreciated their support in my time of need.

The hospital in Osan didn't have CAT scan capabilities, so I was taken by ambulance to Yongson Army hospital, approximately one hour away. The bumpy ride with two chest tubes in place and a portable suction unit would prove to be an unexplainable event commonly referred to as a miracle, which would further strengthen my faith. The ride to the hospital was fairly insignificant except for the malfunction of the portable suction attached to the chest tube. I arrived at Yongson hospital safely and successfully completed the CAT scan procedure.

During the drive home it started to snow, quickly becoming an intense winter storm, causing white out emergency road conditions. The blizzard prompted law enforcement to close the roads to all except emergency vehicles and they could travel no faster than 5 – 10 MPH due to zero visibility. The medical technician and I began to hear a strange noise like I was breathing in a barrel or a hole, and I was becoming progressively short of breath. He thought it was because of the inoperable suction and increased my oxygen to four liters. We checked the chest tubes and could not see anything significant. I remember the panic I felt as I gasped for breath while trying to yell for the technician to call my doctor and tell him to be waiting because I could not breathe. Up in the glass cabinet in the ambulance, I saw something strange. I had thought it was the wings of my guardian angel and began to relax. I kept hearing the words "relax, don't panic, relax." After three hours of moving at a snail's pace, we arrived at Osan hospital where the nurse immediately realized something was wrong and ripped off my blanket to find one of the chest tubes partially disconnected. It was reconnected and attached up to the wall suction and I could breath again instantly. The surgeon ran in and I remember him looking at me saying, "You have a lot of faith." The terrible noise we had heard in the ambulance was air trapped in the muscle as my lung collapsed more and more due to the one-way valve on the lower chest tube dislodging. I was fortunate to be alive. A new chest X-ray to check the tube placement revealed the pneumothorax had enlarged, so I was prepared for a medivac to a thoracic surgeon.

# Chapter 5
# Second Surgery with the Army and Narrative Summary

Tripler Army Hospital in Hawaii was the destination. It was decided that one of the chest tubes was not functioning, so it was removed. The next day, I was taken to the runway by ambulance and loaded on to a C-130 by litter, the same one we had practiced with so often during the exercises. I was flown to Japan where I was immediately transferred to a C-141 hospital plane where it was possible to place a chest tube in the air if complications occurred with the other one I had in place. The Nightengale hospital plane was impressive and I had a nurse and med tech taking care of me and making sure the portable suction was working.

The eight-hour medivac into Hawaii was met by an awaiting ambulance, which rushed me to Tripler Army Hospital where the thoracic surgeon was waiting. He was on his way to surgery, and I was sent to my room to get settled before heading to radiology CAT scan where they would evaluate my status. The radiologist discovered I had a midline shift in my chest, which could cause the other lung to collapse, and notified my surgical team who sent two residents out of the operating room to put in an emergency chest tube. When both lungs collapse in this way, it is called a tension pnuemothorax. Apparently, the existing one had slipped into the intercostals space and was no longer functioning. This was the first chest tube that was not placed in the OR, and since the surgeon felt he needed to place it expeditiously, it was extremely painful.

I awoke the next morning, discussed my case with the thoracic surgeon, signed a few documents and was told the surgery would be sometime that morning. An hour later, I was taken to surgery where, through an incision in my back, a section of my right lung was removed and the rest of it scrubbed and attached to the back wall to prevent it from collapsing again. The thoracic surgeon called it a video assisted thoracotomy, right apical wedge and pleurodesis. After a couple of days and great medications, I began to heal and feel better, until the seventh day when I began to feel pain on the lower right and nausea, which led to a vomiting spell. The X-ray was negative, but I knew something was wrong. I blamed it on the chest tube possibly causing me to retain post-anesthetic gases. Finally, another CAT scan revealed a pneumothorax at the base of my lung. I will never forget the expression on the doctors face when he came to deliver the news that they had to put in a new chest tube immediately or take me back to surgery. My first thought was that another chest tube hooked up to the wall suction would keep me confined to the room for who knows how long. Then I realized it was either another chest tube or I could possibly die. So another chest tube was placed at the base of my lung for another week. My mother flew out to Hawaii, which seemed to help me rejuvenate and summon up my strength and courage. After I was discharged, we stayed at Hickam AFB where I could be watched as an outpatient for a couple of weeks before being medivaced back to Korea.

**NARRATIVE SUMMARY:**

ADMISSION DATE: 21 Feb 1998 1106
DISCHARGE DATE: 09 Mar 1998

1. PRINCIPAL DIAGNOSIS: THORACICIC ENDOMETRIOSIS
2. OTHER DIAGNOSES:
3. PRINCIPAL PROCEDURE/OPERATION: S/P VATS WITH RIGHT APICAL WEDGE RESECTION AND MECHANICAL PLEURODESIS.
4. OTHER PROCEDURES /OPERATIONS
5. PHYSICIANS DISCHARGE NOTE: 41YO FEMALE WITH HISTORY OF EXTRAPELVIC ENDOMETRIOSIS PRESENTS WITH HEMOPNEUMOTHORAX. PT INITIALLY DEVELOPED RIGHT SIDED CHEST PAIN ON 3 FEB 1998. A CXR WAS DONE WHICH DEMONSTRATED RIGHT SIDED PNUEMOTHORAX. PT WAS ADMITTED BY GENERAL SURGERY IN KOREA AND A CHEST TUBE WAS PLACED. A F/U CT SCAN WAS DONE ON 10 FEB WHICH DEMONSTRATED A PNUEMOTHORAX AND CHANGES IN THE CHEST CONSISTENT WITH ENDOMETRIOSIS ACCORDING TO PATIENTS' NARRATIVE SUMMARY FROM KOREA. PT WAS THE MEDIVACED TO TRIPLER AMC FOR FURTHER EVALUATION. PT WAS ADMITTED ON 21 FEB 1998 WHERE SHE UNDERWENT A VATS

PROCEDURE WITH RIGHT APICAL WEDGE RESECTION OF THE LUNG AND MECHANICAL PLEURODESIS. THE OPERATIVE COURSE WAS UNCOMPLICATED. THE PATHOLOGY FROM SURGERY DEMONSTRATED FIBROTIC TISSUE ONLY. NO ENDOMETROSIS. POSTOPERATIVELY, PT EFFUSION PERSISTED AND A PTX DEVELOPED WHICH WAS NOT RELIEVED BY THE PRESENT CHEST TUBE. A CT SCAN WAS DONE ON 1 MARCH WHICH DEMONSTRATED THAT THE PRESENT CHEST TUBE WAS NOT LOCATED IN AN AREA WHICH COULD DRAIN THE EFFUSION AND RELIEVE THE PNUEMOTHORAX. A NEW CHEST TUBE WAS PLACED ON 2 MARCH WHICH RELIEVED THE PNUEMOTHORAX AND CXR CONFIRMED AN EXPANDED LUNG. THE CHEST TUBE WAS KEPT ON SUCTION FOR SEVERAL DAYS AND EVENTUALLY PUT TO WATER SEAL. SERIAL CXRS SHOWED NO EVIDENCE OF PNUEMOTHORAX. THE CHEST TUBE WAS REMOVED ON POD 10 WITHOUT COMPLICATIONS. DURING PATIENT'S HOSPITAL STAY, OB-GYN WAS CONSULTED AND

THEY RECOMMENDED A BONE DENSITY SCAN TO EVALUATE FOR OSTEOPOROTIC CHANGES PRIOR TO POSSIBLY STARTING LUPRON DEPOT THERAPY. PT WILL CONTINUE OCPS UNTIL THEN. PT WILL F/U WITH OB/GYN AS AN OUTPATIENT. PT WAS DISCHARGED ON POD11.

6. DISCHARGE TO HOME

Although I had a lot of pain, to enhance the healing effect and recuperation time, my mother obtained a wheel chair and insisted we go out shopping and tour the island. It was beautiful and I was happy to be alive. My mother left the following week for Texas, and it was time for me to return to Korea. The return medivac was quite different; there were no liters, and thank God I did not need one. We flew to Japan and stayed overnight in a medivac transition clinic before flying on to Korea the next day. Upon entering the small clinic, they asked if I would need to speak to a physician that night. Of course after all I had been through, I said I would absolutely not, but because they were so intrigued with the diagnosis of pulmonary endometriosis they came in to chat at 2:00 am.

I was on convalescent leave for two weeks mainly because of the narcotics I was taking and resumed my military duties after discontinuing them. I had a great commander who insisted I get back in the saddle again before leaving Korea.

It was late March and I was scheduled to a permanent change of station (PCS) back to the United States at Nellis AFB in Las Vegas, Nevada on April 30, 1998. I arrived at Nellis in May 1998 after a fourteen-hour flight from Korea. This time I would be stationed at a hospital with all specialties, which included a pulmonologist. Mike O'Callaghan Federal Hospital was a joint venture with the Veterans Administration and the Air Force. Within a couple of months after arriving at Nellis AFB, my commander discussed placing me on mobility because of the experience I had obtained in Korea. This of course would require a physical and medical release. I scheduled an appointment with the pulmonologist, who was amazed that a medical board was not initiated under the extreme circumstances associated with my condition. After consulting with Wilford Hall, the Air Force major medical center, it was suggested I be placed on a limited profile, which did not include mobility, but did include a watch for six months. There weren't any recurrences during that period and GYN was consulted to recommend extended long term treatment, determined to be birth control pills—Ortho Novum 1/35. Since BC pills had controlled the endometriosis for seven years, they were thought to be the best course of treatment. A full year went by where I participated in gas-mask training and maintained a regular work schedule, treating 8–10 patients per day on average.

I enjoyed living in Las Vegas with unlimited entertainment in the casinos, which I frequented often with many friends and relatives. My health improved and I felt great, although I always felt pressure in the area of the last tube. One year later in May 1999 I was placed on mobility, which meant I was susceptible to deployment, and at Nellis, one of the Air Combat Command bases, it was inevitable.

# Chapter 6
# The Real Test

In August 1999, I received orders for a deployment to Egypt. This was to occur in September 1999 for 90 days. Preparation began and my pulmonologist instructed me to make us proud when he signed my release, and I had every intention of doing so. My gear consisted of a mobility bag, which I would carry on my back, real-world chem gear and a personal bag for a total weight of about fifty pounds. This would be a real test as to whether or not my lung was scarred down, a term frequently used by my thoracic surgeon, which meant not subject to collapse.

The time to leave approached quickly and we were soon on the runway, flying toward our destination. We arrived in Egypt on my birthday, September 12, 1999, and after unloading our gear were told our sleeping tents were ready so we could pick up cots and move in. The following day was a big one because the medical staff put the hospital tents up, which fascinated me. The tents were air-conditioned, insulated, had electricity and even computers and email capability. I discovered there were shower tents and bathroom tents with flushable toilets. This showed how amazing and thoughtful the military was to provide all the amenities of home to make our deployment as comfortable as possible. We put up the hospital the next day and my assistant and I organized the portable dental clinic. I helped move items in and worked hard all day with my colleagues. It took us a couple of days before we were ready to see patients. The patients I treated were multinational and from all branches of service: Army, Air Force, Marines, British, French, Italian and Egyptian.

What an incredible experience it was to have the opportunity to go off base and visit the pyramids and sphinx; it was the icing on the cake. The shopping, my favorite pastime, was also a great distraction in our free time. I met many new people, my health was good and everything seemed to be going fairly well. But one night during a bomb scare as we were being moved closer to the M-60 gun, I tripped over a telephone pole and hit my chest. It knocked the wind out of me, but I thought I would be okay since I could still breathe without any complications. One day while taking down tents, I felt pressure in my right shoulder and it slipped out of its socket. An orthopedic surgeon who was part of our team suggested I have it scoped once we returned to home base. I continued to feel the pain in my shoulder and my blood pressure began to elevate slightly.

Our deployment ended and we had to fly over thirty hours to drop off soldiers and airmen before arriving at Nellis AFB. I felt a little pressure in my chest, but nothing intolerable. Upon arriving at Nevada, I was told we would be given a week off, which I thought would give me time to recuperate. A week later the orthopedic surgeon contacted me to have an X-ray taken of my shoulder, which revealed 700 cc of fluid on my right lung. My pulmonologist ordered a CAT scan and diagnosed me with a loculated hemopnuemothorax. A thoracic surgeon along with GYN was called in for a consult. Since I was not in any immediate distress, it was agreed to administer 3.75 mg of Lupron Depot to attempt resolution of the fluid. After ten days the cat scan was repeated and the fluid started to resolve. In twenty days, most of the fluid was gone and the pulmonologist and thoracic surgeon were happy with the results. My first medical board, which could have resulted in my discharge from the AF, was initiated January 2000. Because of the miraculous results, I was returned to full duty without limitations by decision of the medical command. I was very happy about this decision since I had decided to go back to South Korea for another tour of duty. All the fluid disappeared and GYN decided I would continue on the Lupron Depot, one injection every four months.

Lupron Depot is an interesting medication, initially used to treat prostate cancer, then endometriosis and precocious puberty. My most severe side effect was hot flashes, which I controlled with soy isoflavins. Weight gain was another annoying side effect but my health was good.

In May 2000, I had a PCS back to Osan, South Korea, which gave me the chance to enjoy the Korean culture and finish the incredible shopping experience that makes Korea so unique. Things were great until I put on the gas mask for the fit test. I felt pressure on the right side my neck and that familiar shoulder pain. But this time I tasted a little blood (hemoptisis), which really scared me. I went back to the hospital to see my primary care physician. He could not believe I was allowed to return to Korea, and although there was no fluid on my lung, he recognized the serious consequences that could occur. He set up an immediate consultation with a pulmonologist to evaluate whether my condition was conducive to wearing a gas mask. He also discovered I had not been cleared to fly by my pulmonologist since my last lung-collapsing episode.

For the next two months, all the civilian pulmonologists on the South Korean peninsula were on strike, and we did not have a military lung specialist stationed in Korea. My family practice physician decided I should be medivaced back to Hawaii to see a pulmonologist and my thoracic surgeon to determine if the gas mask could be worn in the future and to clear me to fly, which I thought was ridiculous since I flew fourteen hours into Korea. I was a little nervous about the hemoptisis, so I agreed. This medivac was to occur one week before my pediatric continuing education course in San Antonio, Texas. I wasn't aware my doctor thought I would never return to Korea and my objective was to get cleared to fly and make it to my course.

I flew in to Hawaii September 2000 and saw the pulmonologist the next day. Since pulmonary endometriosis is so rare, he could not determine whether I could wear the gas mask or not and referred me to the thoracic surgeon who performed the surgery in 1998, since it was his handy work. The surgeon remembered me and was shocked my lung had collapsed again, but decided subsequent events could occur even though presently my lung appeared scarred down. I was cleared to fly on commercial airlines pressurized at 8000 to 10,000 feet. He did not feel the gas mask was conducive to good lung function, but could not see any blebs on X-ray that could be causing hemoptosis.

Well, since I had been cleared to fly and had orders to go to San Antonio, Texas, I jumped in a taxi and headed for Hickam AFB Sato Travel. They issued me a plane ticket, and I left the next day for the two-week pediatric dental course, which was extremely informative. I left there and flew to Midland for one week to visit my mother, then returned to Korea. My physician was waiting and extremely surprised I attended the CE course.

A second medical board convened immediately. It was now October and maybe taking Lupron Depot every four months was working. In December, I developed pressure in my chest and the X-ray revealed fluid. Three consecutive months of Lupron Depot had been required to resolve it. The board returned with a decision to send me back to the United States and restrict me with what is called a C-code, meaning I can only serve on active duty in the United States. The decision had been made, but I was allowed to finish my tour and return to the U.S. in May. My original orders for the next tour were to go to Misawa, Japan but were changed to Los Angeles AFB. Since I grew up in LA, I was happy with the decision. I had thought I would stay for a year perhaps and maybe go into private practice. But before this would all take place, I still had four months to enjoy Korea, which included extensive shopping trips and seeing everything I missed during my first tour.

I worked a normal-duty day and during the exercises was assigned to processing detail or treating emergency patients. My tour ended without a significant incidence and I arrived at Los Angeles AFB 29 May 2001 to start my last tour of duty. Fort MacArthur in San Pedro, CA was my temporary home for five days and then it was on to the Budget 9 Motel in Redondo Beach for two months while my townhouse cleared escrow. I started my daily routine of treating patients in the clinic and assumed my military duties.

To continue care with a pulmonologist, I was sent to the Navy Medical Center in Balboa, 124 miles from Los Angeles. It was explained that I had to be treated in a military facility unless it was an emergency because it was a fit-for-duty issue. My new Navy pulmonologist referred me to a specialist in GYN who stressed the severity of my disease and the need for a hysterectomy. I informed her surgery would be difficult because the base of my lung would possibly collapse, plunging us into an unwanted situation. We spent the next year with visits every three months to check for fluid and to talk about surgery. In December 2001, I developed pressure on the right side and was placed on Lupron Depot throughout January, February, and March. X-rays revealed the fluid had resolved. There are no safe studies for the use of Lupron Depot for more than a six-month interval.

# Chapter 7

# Third Surgery With the Navy and Narrative Summary

May 16 (Thursday) while running for a mock code blue exercise at Los Angeles Air Force Base, I noticed I was getting short of breath. I was scheduled off on Friday and Monday was a holiday. On Saturday I began to hear a slight wheezing sound and the shortness of breath continued, but I thought with a little rest I would be fine. On Tuesday my symptoms had not changed, so I went to sick call where a chest X-ray was taken. Because my pneumothorax was loculated, the primary care physician determined it to be normal and breath sounds could be heard on that side. I knew something wrong was causing my shortness of breath and I felt I needed Lupron Depot right away, which the pharmacy at LAAFB did not stock. I was allowed to drive to San Diego, taking the X-ray with me to see my GYN doc for a shot of Lupron Depot. She read the first report, gave me 3.75 mg of IM Lupron Depot, listened for breath sounds, checked the X-ray and scheduled a follow-up appointment.

I returned to work the next day, Tuesday 21 August and continued treating patients until 28 August. I became so short of breath I could not prescribe medication for my patient. I ran down to primary care where another X-ray was taken, revealing a slight midline shift. The doctor on duty knew instantly what had happened and she heard dull breath sounds on the lower right, indicating a possible pneumothorax. My pulmonologist was contacted and his staff gave me an appointment for the next day or emergency room if urgent. It took a lot of convincing, but finally the doc agreed to allow me to drive myself to see the pulmonologist. I had the SOS in my car and they would send emergency vehicles to my location if needed, so I felt fairly confident. I phoned my GYN doc that evening to inform her I was coming in the next day and she suggested I pack a small bag for a possible overnight stay. I sat up in bed to sleep that night because I was so short of breath.

The drive to San Diego the next day seemed longer than usual and I had a lot of anxiety.

Within an hour of seeing the pulmonologist, I had the first painless chest tube placed by the radiology department and was admitted to the hospital. The chest tube was placed while I was awake with lidocaine around the incision area. My pulmonologist informed me he would be leaving the next day for a permanent change of duty to Florida. The next day, 30 May 2002, as I watched my pulse oximeter drop from 99 to 85, pressure developed against my trachea, cutting off my ability to swallow and completely shutting off my breathing ability. The nurse had entered the room and ran to get the residents. Within minutes my room was filled with people not sure what was happening when a miracle occurred. My pulmonologist walked into my room to say goodbye before leaving for Florida but, read the apparent symptoms and immediately went into action. He pulled my chest tube apart and took a 20 cc syringe, pulling the air out twice and decompressing my chest to cause my lung to pop back into place. I was extremely grateful my guardian angel showed up with impeccable timing. He cleared the chest tube with saline, discovering the tension pneumothorax occurred because it was clogged. That was our last encounter. The chest tube was hooked up to the wall suction and the rest of the day was insignificant. A larger chest tube was placed when the X-ray revealed significant fluid build up the next day.

The next few days of fluid increase influenced a GYN and pulmonology decision toward a hysterectomy with bilateral salpingo oopherectomy (removal of both ovaries). Cardiothoracic surgery consulted regarding another pleurodisis, but GYN won and surgery was scheduled. I would be awake during the surgery with an epidural for pain control and the chest tube would be left in. It was also explained that if there were any problems during the surgery, I would have to be placed on a ventilator—one of my worst fears.

I was taken to surgery Monday June 3 and thankfully there were no complications. The epidural was left in for three days, so I had no postoperative surgical pain from the hysterectomy, but a sharp, unbearable pain occurred on the left side so severely I was given morphine. A CAT scan revealed fluid on my left lung due to possible damage occurring during the tension pneumothorax. My hematocrit/hemoglobin dropped to critical levels and two units of blood were transfused. Instead of getting better I seem to be getting worse. I spiked a temperature and a bacterium was found in my blood. The epidural and chest tube was removed and I was started on antibiotics. I was beginning to feel better and my blood count increased. I was told I could go home but would have to be treated with an IV of a very strong antibiotic called Timentin for three weeks. I agreed, a PICC line was placed, Lupron Depot was given IM and I was assigned a home health-care nurse and discharged. I continued to improve with no other treatment required except monthly injections of Lupron Depot until September 13.

## NAVY NARRATIVE SUMMARY FOR MEDICAL BOARD

MAJ GLYNIS WALLACE IS FOLLOWED BY PULMONARY CLINIC FOR PULMONARY ENDOMETRIOSIS. THIS WAS FIRST DIAGNOSED IN 1991, AND THE PATENT HAS UNDERGONE MULTIPLE PROCEDURES FOR THIS DIAGNOSIS INCLUDING MULTIPLE CHEST TUBE PLACEMENT AND VIDEO-ASSISTED THORACOSCOPY WITH WEDGE RESECTION.

SHE, MOST RECENTLY, WAS ADMITTED TO THE INPATIENT MEDICINE SERVICE AT NAVAL MEDICAL CENTER SAN DIEGO ON 29 MAY 2002 WITH COMPLAINT OF DYSPNEA AND EVIDENCE OF A RECURRENT PNERMOTHORAX ON CHEST X-RAY. SHE HAD PREVIOUSLY BEEN TREATED WITH

LUPRON DEPOT THERAPY APPROXIMATELY THREE MONTHS PRIOR TO ADMISSION. SHE WAS TREATED WITH PIGTAIL CATHETER DRAINAGE. HER COURSE WAS COMPLICATED BY RECURRENCE OF A TENTION PNEUMOTHORAX WHEN THE CHEST TUBE BECAME CLOGGED. THIS WAS RESOLVED WITHOUT DIFFUCULTY AND HER LUNGS REEXPANDED FULLY.

DURING THAT ADMISSION, SHE UNDER WENT A TOTAL ABDOMINAL HYSTERECTOMY WITH BILATERAL SALPINGO-OOPHORECTOMY. SHE TOLERATED THE PROCEDURE WELL. THE COURSE WAS COMPLICATED BY REQUIREMENT FOR TRANSFUSION OF TWO UNITS OF PACKED RED BLOOD CELLS, A SMALL LEFT PLEURAL EFFUSION AND URINARY TRACT INFECTION WITH E. COLI AND ENTEROCOCCUS. SHE HAD PERSISTENT FEVER, AND BLOOD CULTURES GREW BACTEROIDES SPECIES, AND THE PATIENT WAS TREATED WITH A PROLONGED COURSE OF TIMENTIN. SHE WAS DISCHARGED ON 13 JUNE 2002.

AT THIS TIME, SHE HAS UNDERGONE DEFINITIVE THERAPY FOR HER EXTRAPELVIC ENDOMETRIOSIS. SHE OBVIOUSLY WILL HAVE CONTINUED

SERUM ESTROGEN LEVELS IN THE POSTMEOPAUSAL RANGE DUE TO PERIPHERAL CONVERSION OF ESTROGEN, ADIPOSE TISSUE AND PROBABLY ENDOMETRIAL IMPLANTS AS WELL. THE CLINICAL SIGNIFICANCE OF THIS PERSISTENT ESTROGEN LEVEL IS UNCERTAIN. IN MANY CASES REPORTED IN THE LITERATURE, PATIENTS WHO WERE TREATED MEDICALLY AND HAD SYMPTOMS FROM ESTROGEN SUPRESSION WERE TREATED WITH LOW DOSE OF EXTROGEN THERAPY WITHOUT RECURRENCE OF PNEUMOTHORAX. ADDITIONALLY, ORAL CONTRACEPTIVES ARE A FIRST LINE THERAPY FOR CATAMENIAL PNU\EMOTHORAX AND PLEURAL ENDOMETRIOSIS. THEREFORE, I FEEL THAT MAJ WALLACE'S RISK FOR RECURRENT PNUEMOTHORAX IS LOW; HOWEVER I CONNOT EXCLUDE THAT IT MAY HAPPEN AGAIN IN THE FUTURE.

# Chapter 8
# No Cure

I was given the Lupron Depot after surgery because the only definitive cure for endometriosis is surgical resection or complete destruction of the endometriotic lesion. I would have to have more thoracic surgery to remove the implants on my lung, which I did not consider a viable option at this point. All literature currently available on the subject stated surgical management does not include bilateral salpingo-oophorectomy. Removal of the ovaries will not ensure relief of symptoms because estrogen is also produced by peripheral conversion of androgens (primarily androstenedione of adrenal and ovarian origin). This conversion is catalyzed by aromatase. Aberrant aromatase expression has been identified in edometriotic, implants causing local production of estradiol within the implant. (Noble et al, 1996). I started collecting research on catamenial pneumothoracies from all over the world—the United Kingdom, Japan, etc.—because I desperately wanted a cure; however, my search confirmed the existing information.

I went back to work the last week in August and found it difficult treating patients 8–10 hours a day, so I was given a limited work day. A medical board was initiated to decide fitness for duty, which culminated into a medical separation from the United States Air Force on December 22, 2002.

## AIR FORCE MEDICAL BOARD SUMMARY:

INTRODUCTION: Glynis Wallace, is a 45 y/o active duty Air Force Major who has been under the care of LAAFB since her PCS from Osan AFB in May 2001 for pulmonary endometriosis.

HPI: Major Wallace is an active duty Air Force dentist who presented to our clinic for follow-up on pulmonary endometriosis. An MEB was done in Oct 2000 with return to duty with a Code C limitation. Major Wallace was doing well on Lupron Depot, being followed by Gynecology at NMC. She began to experience persistent shortness of breath 28 May 02 and was referred and subsequently admitted to NMC 29 May 02 with right hemopneumothorax. A CT guided pigtail catheter was inserted with full re-expansion of the right lung. On the second hospital day, a right sided tension Pneumothorax developed secondary to clog in the chest tube, which resolved with a change to a larger chest tube and wall suction for 24 hours, then water seal. On 3 June 02 she underwent modified radical hysterectomy with bilateral salpingo oophorectomy. On post-op day 2(POD #2), she developed symptomatic anemia and was transfused with 2 units PRBCs. Also on POD #2, she developed recurrent Pneumothorax which resolved with chest tube placed to wall suction, then to water seal. The chest tube was removed on POD #4. Major Wallace developed a fever of 102.7 post-op with a subsequent urine culture positive for E. coli and Enterococcus with treatment with Ampicillin, Gentamycin and Flagy.Blood cultures were also positive for bacteroides with a change of antibiotics to Timentin. A PICC line was inserted prior to discharge on 13 June 02 for home IV Timentin therapy for 3 weeks. A left sided pleural effusion was noted on CRX done during hospitalization, which resolved spontaneously. However,

Major Wallace continues to be evaluated by Ob/Gyn and Pulmonology at NMC, with her next appointments being 13 Sep 02.

PAST MEDICAL HISTORY: Abdominal and thoracic endometrial disease, diagnosed in 1991 after presenting with ascites and right pleural effusion. She was treated with primary resection of the colonic Endometrial disease and hormonal regulation of her thoracic disease. In Feb 1998 she was treated for hemopneumothorax of the right chest with multiple chest tubes and a wedge resection with video assisted thoracic surgery (VATS). Major Wallace has had 2 further episodes of hemopneumothorax in Dec 1999 and Dec 2000.

PAST SURGICAL HISTORY:
Colonic resection of Endometrial disease 1991

Wedge resection with VATS right lung 1998

Chest tube placement1991, Feb and March 1998, May 2002

Abdominal hysterectomy with bilateral salpingo oophrectomy June 2002

MEDICATIONS:
Lupron Depot once a month for 6 months
Celebrex 200 mg BID
Calcium

ALLERGIES
NKDA

HABITS:
No tobacco use

PHYSICAL EXAM
General: NAD, Alert and oriented x 4, WD/WN

HEENT:NC/AT, PERRLA, EOMI, O/P clear, TMs intact Lungs: CTAB

Heart: RRR, no murmur

Abdomen: + BS x 4, NT, ND, No HSM. Well healed abdominal scar

Ext: No CCE, 2 +pulses bilaterally

CONSULTATIONS: Major Wallace was previously seen by a cardiothoracic surgeon, at Tripler Army Medical Center. His assessment was that she had recurrent hemopnuemothoraces, and that subsequent events may occur, and are unpredictable.

LABS AND STUDIES:
CXR 8/8/02: right apical bullae. Fibrotic band right upper/lower lung. Blunting of right costophrenic angle, possible fibrosis

CBC 8/8/02: HGB 12.9/HCT 38.

ASSESSMENT: Pulmonary endometriosis with recurrent hemopneumothoraces requiring multiple chest tube placements, s/p abdominal hysterectomy with bilateral salpingo oophrectomy, currently managed on Lupron Depot therapy once a month

LINE OF DUTY: Yes

WWQ: No

PROFILE: 4C Oct 00

MILITARY IMPAIRMENT: Dr Wallace is able to perform all duties as an Air Force dentist. She is unable to participate in military exercises and wear chemical protective mask.

DISPOSITION AND/OR RECOMMENDATIONS:
Major Wallace has a chronic disease currently controlled with monthly Lupron Depot therapy. However, considering the unpredictability of

pulmonary endometriosis, she needs to be stationed in a locale with access to tertiary level of medical care for a period of up to 2 years. Being stationed at a remote location with high operation tempo would put Major Wallace's health and life at risk. Major Wallace has requested separation from military service. Support to this decision is justified considering the possibility of hemopneumothorax recurrence and the severity of the last occurrence.

The civilian phase of dealing with this unknown disease began with a trip to the veteran's hospital. Of course the doctors have never heard of it and are not sure how to treat it. It's critical for me to convey all information necessary for them to keep me alive. I knew I had to write this book because it could possibly help save my life.

The Veterans Administration would now administer my medical care. The shocked looks and disbelief would start all over again, along with the uncertainty as to how to proceed with treatment.

My first visit was as expected. It was decided we would treat symptoms as they arose with a preventive chest X-ray initiated by the pulmonary department every six months. Fear drove me to the emergency room with pain radiation down my right side. An X-ray and CAT scan reassured me my lung had not collapsed on the right side and it was possibly adhesions from my chest tubes. I was relieved and decided to stop living my life as though I was waiting for the next episode to occur. Immediately after making that decision, fate arrive to help me and a wonderful opportunity appeared. I would start my very own dental practice and pay the military back by offering a 10% discount to everyone with military affiliation. Once the plan was initiated, it was unstoppable.

After locating a place and securing the lease, redirecting my focus and energy caused me to become too busy to think about illness or my disease. The excitement of starting my very own business was just the adrenalin rush I needed to make me want to get up early, stay up late and focus on a positive outcome. I opened the practice June 2003 and the military members were there to take care of me once again by helping me build my practice.

A week after starting the practice, I met the love of my life—a kind, understanding, non-judgmental man who gave me unconditional love. He was a former marine who served in the Vietnam War, so he understood the military. We were married April 2004. He works hard at trying to understand the disease and does whatever he can to help.

The six-month preventive chest X-rays remain clear and the incentive spirometer seems to keep my lung volume fairly stable.

# References

1. Roberts LM, Redan J, Reich H. Extraperitoneal Endometriosis, Catamenial Pneumothoracies, And Review of the Literature. The Trocar :: Online Videojournal of Gynecologic and Surgical Endoscopy 2002.

2. Perrotin C, Mussot S, Fadel E, Chapelier A, DartvelleP. Catamenial Pneumothorax. Failure of videothorascopic treatment. Presse Med 2002 Mar 9;31(9): 402-4 (Medline)

3. Yokoyama T, Tomoda M, Kanbara T, Nishiyama T, Manabe M. Epidural anesthesia for patient with catamenial pneumothorax. Masui 2001 Mar; 50(3):290-2 (Medline)

4. Tsunezuka Y, Sato H, Kodama T, Shimizu H, Kurumaya H. Expression of CA125 in thoracic endometriosis in a patient with catamenial pneumothorax. Respiration 1999; 66(5):470-2 (Medline)

5. Noble LS, Simpson ER, Johns A, et al. Aromatase expression in endometriosis. J Clin Endocrinol Metab 1996; 81: 174-179. (Medline)

6. Schoenfeld A, Ziv E, Aeelel Y, et al, Catamenial Pneumothorax: a literature review and report of and unusual case. Obstet Gynecol Surv 1986; 41:20-24. (Medline)

7. Foster DC, Stern JL, Buscema J, et al. Pleural and parenchymal pulmonary endometriosis. Obstet Gynecol 1981; 58:552-556. (Medline)

8. Rossi NP and Goplerud CP. Recurrent catamenial Pneumothorax. Arch Surg 1974; 109:173-176. (Medline)

9. Lillington GA, Mitchell SP, Wood GA. Catamenial Pneumothorax. JAMA 1972; 219:1328-1332. (Medline)

10. Crutcher RR, Waltuch TL, Blue ME. Recurrent spontaneous Pneumothorax associated with menstruation. J Thorac Cardiovasc Surg 1967; 54: 599-602. (Medline)

11. Maurer ER, Schaal JA, Mendex FL. Chronic recurring spontaneous Pneumothorax due to endometriosis of the diaphragm. JAMA 1958: 168: 2013-2014.

Printed in the United States
77159LV00001B